Nail Art

Easy, Glamorous and Inspiring DIY Nail Art Designs for Your Fingers & Toes

1st Edition

By Francine Agile

Under no circumstances will any legal responsibility or blame be held against the publisher for any reparation, damages, or monetary loss due to the information herein, either directly or indirectly.

Respective authors own all copyrights not held by the publisher.

The information herein is offered for informational purposes solely, and is universal as so. The presentation of the information is without contract or any type of guarantee assurance.

The trademarks that are used are without any consent, and the publication of the trademark is without permission or backing by the trademark owner. All trademarks and brands within this book are for clarifying purposes only and are the owned by the owners themselves, not affiliated with this document.

Table of Contents

Chapter 1: History of Nail Art

Have you ever seen very detailed and beautiful nails? How did people come up with this kind of art, anyway? Nail art actually started several thousands of years ago, with very basic designs and materials until certain people found new ways to make nail art easier and more glamorous. Below is the timeline on how nail art progressed to what it is today:

- The first nail treatment can be traced back in 5000 B.C. when women from Ancient Egypt dyed their nails with henna to symbolize their status.
- In 3200 B.C., men from Babylon were also painting their nails. Believe it or not, the activity is a part of their preparation for war, in their hopes that these would make them more fearsome.

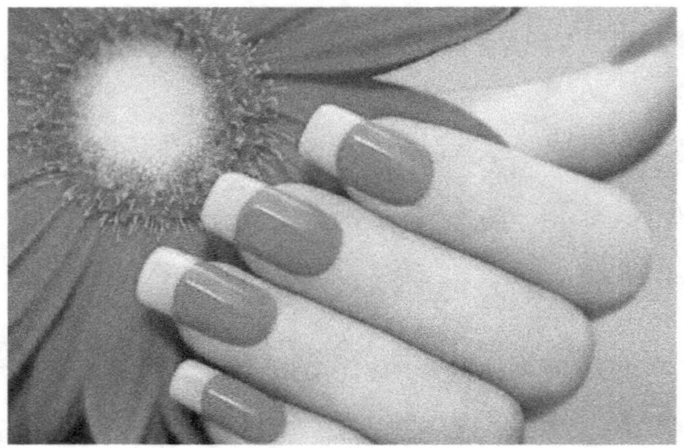

- Approximately two hundred years later and human civilization discovered the first nail polish. Women in Ancient China mixed gelatin, egg whites, vegetable dyes, gum Arabic and beeswax but the process was very tedious as it required women to dip their nails in the mixture for several hours.

- Then in the 15th century, during the Incan Empire, a large civilization in South America, the Incas started to experiment more on their nails by painting eagles on them.

- In 1770, gold and silver manicure sets were made – an invention that was definitely fit for a king, since French King Louis XVI had used these sets until his deposition in 1792.

- It was in the 18th century when materials for nail treatment have progressed from acid, scissors and metal rod to include the orange wooden stick invented by Dr. Sitts, a European podiatrist.

- In 1907, the first liquid nail polish was created and soon, a variety of colors was available for nail decoration.

- Just a few years later, in 1925, the Lunar manicure or the Half-Moon manicure became a trend.

The Half-Moon manicure will be discussed further in Chapter Seven: Nail Art Ideas and Designs for Beginners. Since then, even celebrities have either started or joined the trend of wearing exotic nail art designs.

Chapter 2: What is Nail Art

But what is nail art, anyway? Simply put, nail art is an activity of designing one's fingernails and toenails. The design could be a fashion statement, a form of expression or a little bit of both.

Nail art is most commonly considered a fashion statement, though, depending on a person's choice, the design of one's fingernails and/ or toenails could match with a person's whole outfit or it could also go against the flow, such as in the case of accent nails, which are manicured or pedicured nails with a different design than the rest of the remaining nails on a hand or foot.

On another hand, nail art could also be a form of expression as it was in history wherein nail design could hold a deeper meaning. In fact, in 2016, the Polished Man challenge was issued to several Hollywood actors such as Chris

Hemsworth, Hugh Jackman and Zac Effron. Some of these actors have painted one of their nails to show their support in raising awareness to children who have suffered from physical and emotional violence.

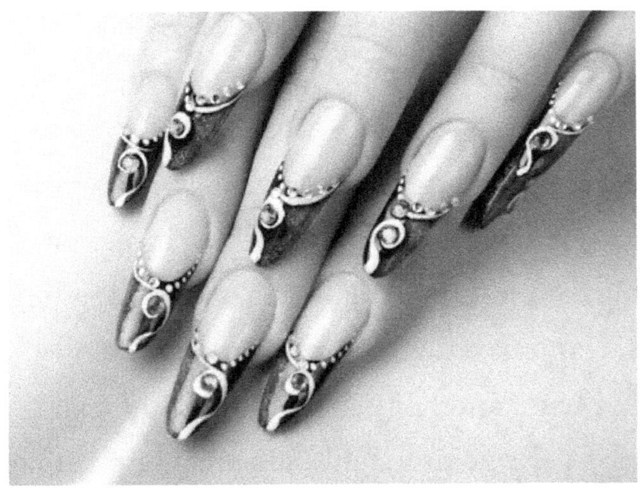

Chapter 3: Why Have Nail Art?

The reasons why people indulged in nail art could include the following:

- **To express creativity.** With the various designs that the people have sported and the different materials and tools available, a person can be as creative as possible.

- **To use it as a form of relaxation or for the pursuit of happiness.** People have found happiness, or at least relaxation, while designing nails. Happiness and relaxation can also be found even if another person is doing the nail art for a person; although some might argue that satisfaction may be a bit toned down in this case.

- **To go with the trend or the latest fashion statement.**

- **To stand up for a cause.** As is the Polished Man challenge mentioned in the previous chapter.

- **To hide nail imperfections.** Wouldn't it be so tempting to turn a damaged nail into a glamorous nail? Just beware of chemicals contained in nail art materials to avoid damaging the nail further.

- **To bond with other people.** Nail art could be a great activity together.

The above list is not all inclusive. There may be other reasons that may be unique to you. Who knows? You'll never know what nail art could mean to you unless you try without any reserves.

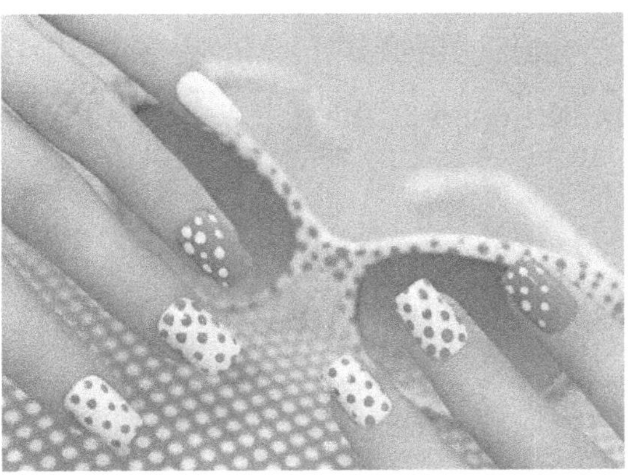

Chapter 4: What's Involved - Materials and Methods

Materials needed depend on the desired design. The following materials are the most basic of all for nail art:

Nail polish.

There are various types of nail enamels, such as staple, neon, nude, metallic, pastel, fluorescent, jewel tone and glitter. Designs can be done even with just nail polish. A combination of it can be used for some simple nail art designs such as the half-moon manicure and the ombre nails. To emphasize the color of the nail polish, add a layer of white nail polish first before applying a layer of the desired type and color of nail polish. This prevents the natural color of the nail to affect the top-most polish.

Just avoid formaldehyde, toluene and resins which are common contact allergens.

Base coats.

Use base coats for the following reasons:

- **Prevent damage to your nails.** Nail polish contains harmful chemicals. Base coats serve as defense from these. For better protection, apply two layers of base coat. Apply the first layer on the upper portion of the nail only and then apply the second layer to the full nail. This is to prevent the tips of the nails from chipping.

If base coat is not going to be used, it is advised to avoid dark and neon colors to prevent nail damage. Nail polish with high-quality and long-lasting formula is also recommended.

- **Prolong your manicure.** Base coats have plasticizers that make them flexible and cellulose chemicals which act as an adhesive to your nail and your polish, which prevent the polish from peeling off.

- **Care for your nails.** The chemicals in a base coat can also address nail problems. There are base coats that are intended for dry nails and there are those as well for nails with uneven surface. Base coats could also strengthen nails. Do not, however, use nail hardeners that contain too much formaldehyde. As advertised, this will harden nails but the formaldehyde can harden them too much to the point that it'll cause them to break, which is very ironic, indeed.

- **Even the texture of nail polish.**
As is the case in nail polish, toluene and resins should also be avoided.

- **Top coats.** With right use, base coats and top coats both prolong the manicure so what is the difference? A nail should have a different base coat and top coat since base coats do not have the shine that is desired in top coats whereas top coats do not have the chemicals that glues the nail polish to the nail bed.

Acrylic nails.

For quick nail art, nail art stickers and acrylic nails may be used. Acrylic nails can be very tempting to use since these nail art designs are immediately available for application. There is also no risk that the design may be different on application than expected since the acrylic nails are only applied on a person's nail plates as is. In addition, acrylic nails may also allow an artist to create more complex designs on the acrylic nails than one's own hand. However, the use of acrylic nails is not really recommended and they should be used with extreme caution. Preferably, these should be applied by professionals. Those interested in acrylic nails should be aware of the possibility that the acrylic nail may not be sufficiently attached to the nail bed during its application.

The space would allow for water to enter and the moisture, warmth and darkness would consequently allow a fungus infection to occur and to thrive. Since acrylic nails may not be removed for months, the infection may remain unseen and untreated. In the worst-case scenario, this may result to the detachment of the nail plate from the nail bed. Treatment of the infection may take six months to a year.

Those interested in acrylic nails are advised that there are other ways to get the design that they want. An improvised procedure will be further discussed in *Chapter 6 How to do Nail Art at Home – Step by Step*.

For do-it-yourself nail art, the following materials could be used, in addition to any or some, if not all, of those that were already mentioned.

- **Transfer Foils.** These give nails a shimmery, one-of-a-kind finish.

- **Striping Tapes.** These thin tapes, with different colors and textures, add straight metallic lines to nails.

- **Loose glitter/ confetti glitter.** For a shimmery effect, apply top coat on nails, dip nails in glitter, remove excess with a fan brush and apply another layer of top coat to seal in the glitters.

To go for 3D nail art, the following materials may be added:

- **Acrylic mixture.** This provides the flexibility needed in drawing different shapes and objects.

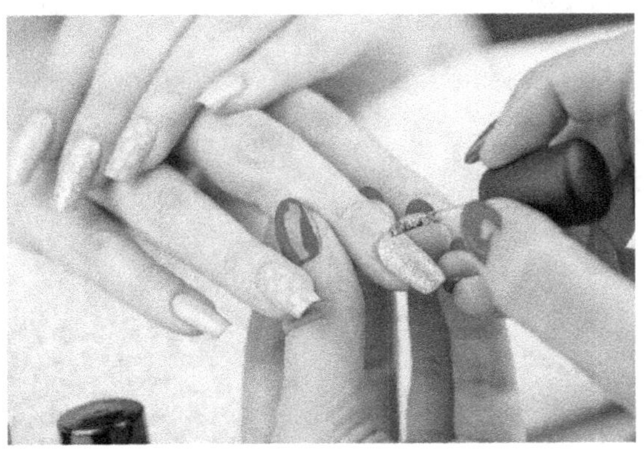

• **Cavier beads/ bullion beads/ sprinkle beads.** These small glass or metal beads create the accent desired in a 3D nail art.

• **Rhinestones, domed pearls, sequins and studs.** These come in different shapes, colors and sizes.

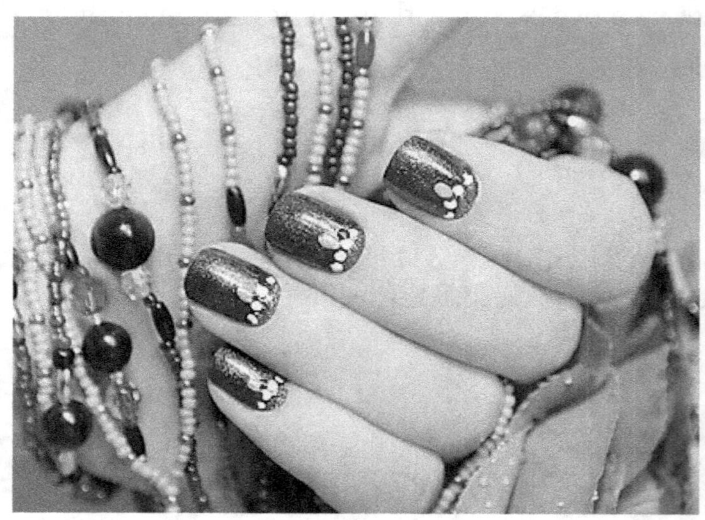

Chapter 5: Nail Art Tools

Most of the materials enumerated in the previous chapters cannot be applied on the nail without nail art tools. These tools are discussed below.

First, the nail has to be cared for using the following tools:

Nail polish remover.

There are various types to choose from: liquid, wipes, correction pen and glitter pads.

The liquid, normal ones are the most common, the easiest and most likely, the cheapest one in the list. It could still be the most effective, depending on how it is used.

 Wipes should also be considered because these:

o   Do not contain alcohol, acetone, toluene and paraben.

o Contain natural olive oil and vitamin E for shiny and healthy-looking nails.

o Easily removes dark nail polish.

o Correction pens can also be very handy in correcting minute details of the nail art.

o Glitter pads can also be considered to avoid frustration in removing glitter nail polish.

Lint-free cotton swabs.

These prevent cotton fibers from ruining the manicure.

Nail repair formula.

Use every once in a while, or as necessary, depending on the frequency and toxicity of the chemicals applied on the nails.

Nail cutter and nail file.

Use these to shape up your nails. The shape of the nails may also be a part of the overall design. Some use these to create pointy nail ends that add to edgy nail designs.

The following tools, on the other hand, are used to apply the designs:

Nail art brushes, including striper brush.

Nail art brushes come in different sizes. One of which is the thin striper brush which help create minute details. The brush does not necessarily have to be purchased or made for the purpose of nail art. Others such as eyebrow brush may be used, as long as their cleanliness can be ensured.

Dotting Tools.

If you want to make fancy nail designs, a dotting tool is a must for any nail art fan. While it's possible to purchase one ready-made for the purpose, it's also extremely simple and cheap (if not free) to make one of your own from items already available in the house. Just quickly Google how to make dotting tools.

Nail Adhesive Glue.

This is used to attach acrylic nail and other materials to the nail plate.

Stamping Kit.

Stamping kits include stamp, scraper and stamping template. It is advised to purchase them separately for more customization and to ensure quality of each tool. Additionally, it may be good to purchase several stamping templates so that there would be at least one template that would suit a chosen theme or design.

The step-by-step guide on how to use these tools can be found in *Chapter Seven: Nail Art Ideas and Designs for Beginners.*

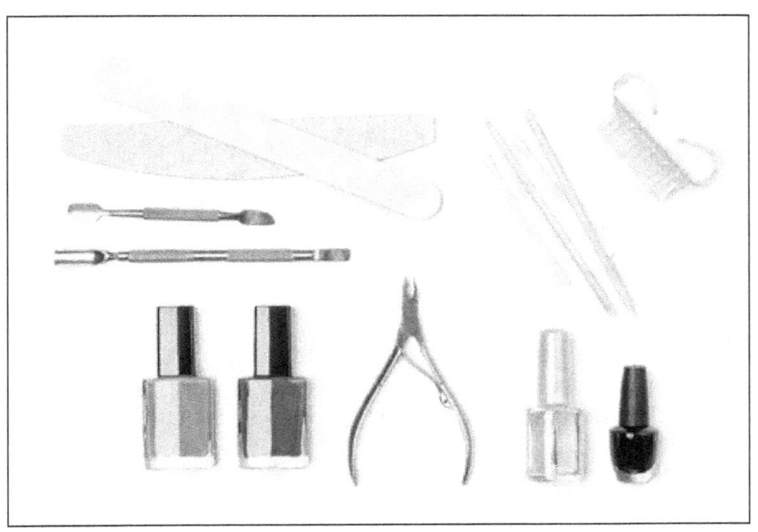

Tweezers.

These are used for picking up 3D materials rhinestones and domed pearls.

Orangewood Stick or Toothpick.

These are used for creating dots, picking rhinestones and water marbling.

Scissors.

These are used to cut decals and other excess materials.

LED Nail Lamp.

Just hold the nail lamp over gel polishes for the nail polish to harden.

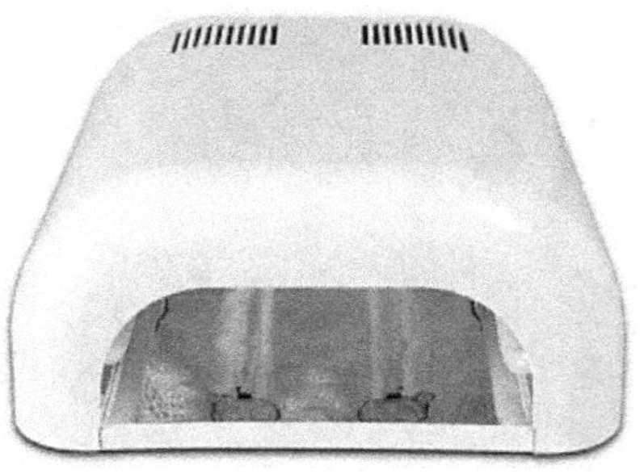

Gel polishes are very convenient to use since they dry instantly and they last long but these are not recommended because they:

- **Cause nail damage**. The use of gel polish may result to nail breakage, thinning and infections. Specialists claim that nails need to recover for weeks due to damage from gel treatment.

- **Pose health risks beyond the nail area.** There were reports that the UV lights used in the gel treatment can lead to cancer.

- **Are tougher to remove.** The method of removing the gel polish (filing them off or soaking them up in acetone) can further damages the nails.

Chapter 6: Nail Art at Home – Step by Step

There are many ways to experiment with nail art at home. Only a very simple and easy way is explained here, and is as follows:

- **Remove old nail polish or nail art.** Use liquid, wipes, correction pen or glitter pads. Other materials may also be needed depending on the nail art to be removed. For acrylic nails, place a small bowl of liquid acetone nail polish remover on a larger bowl with hot water. The hot water outside the small bowl adds heat to the acetone nail polish remover and makes it more effective. Dip the nails in nail polish remover for about five minutes. Then pour baby oil on cotton swab and rub the swab on each nail. Apply it in a circular motion to remove remaining glue and to moisturize the nails. Liberally use the baby oil as the moisturizing effect is much needed after the nails have been subjected to prolonged exposure to acetone.

To remove glittery and other stubborn nail polish, soak cotton in nail polish remover. Place the cotton and wrap the foil around the finger, including the cotton. Leave them on for five minutes and the nail polish will be removed once the cotton and the foil are disposed of.

- **Trim nails.** Better if the design of the nail would go with the shape of the nails. Feminine nail designs are better off with rounded squares, whereas edgy nail designs are good with structural fingertips.

- **Use nail repair formula every now and then or as necessary.**

- **Apply base coat.** Allow this to completely dry before proceeding. To easily remove glitter nail polish, consider using Elmer's glue as base coat.

The use of special base coat might be able to address nail problems such as brittle and/ or dry nails; however, foregoing Elmer's glue might require the nails to be subjected to long exposure to harmful acetone, instead of simply using Elmer's glue to create a more easily-removable nail art.

• **Paint nails.** Also allow this to completely dry before proceeding.

• **Apply top coat.**

More step-by-step guides will be provided per design or idea that will be mentioned in the next two chapters.

If the nail art materials and tools mentioned in the previous chapters are not available, there are other alternatives, in do-it-yourself (DIY) nail art materials and tools.

These are as follows:

- **Petroleum jelly.** Apply petroleum jelly on the surrounding skin of the nail before applying polish for easy clean-up

- **DIY glitter nail polish.** Combine loose glitter/ confetti glitter with plain colored nail polish instead of purchasing new glitter nail polish

- **Regular gel pen.** Use regular gel pen for drawings and minute details, instead of nail art brushes which may be too thick or too hard to control. For a thicker effect, Sharpie pen may be used.

- **Bobby pin.** Use a bobby pin as a dotting tool.

• **Punchers.** Maximize punchers commonly used for artistic purposes, such as punchers with clover-shaped holes. Use them to punch shapes on nail art tapes. Press nail art tapes firmly on nail and apply nail polish over the hole.

And voila for the perfectly-shaped nail polish. Just don't forget to apply top coat after the polish has dried.

• **Band-aid.** Use band-aids for that easy polka dot design. Just press the band-aid firmly on the nail, but not too firmly that it might leave some of the adhesive behind on the nail. Once done, apply nail polish over it. Remove the band-aid and also apply the top coat. Similarly, lace, nets and loofahs may be used to create different designs.

- **Regular tape dispenser.** Use regular tape dispenser for easy storage and use of nail strip tape.

And so on. It is recommended that research is first conducted on the materials and tools that you plan to buy before purchasing anything. Check out reviews from different websites and check contents to look out for harmful chemicals. Also check if there are other DIY alternatives that might just seem a little too improvised but may actually be very economical, efficient and/or creative.

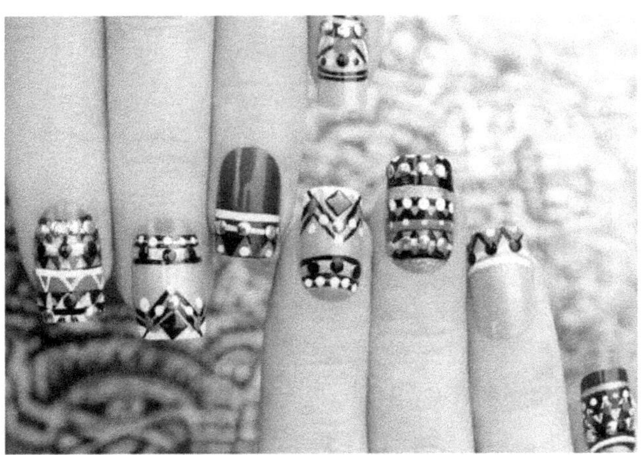

Chapter 7: Nail Art Ideas & designs

There are a lot of methods and styles for you to explore on. The sky is the limit on your design. What's best is that there is no need to apply an experiment on one nail to the rest. Accent nails are quite common and it gives the following advantages:

• It provides relief especially if the design on one nail is too tedious or too prone to error if recreated;

• It is not too demanding on materials, especially if materials would not be sufficient to be applied on all nails; and

• It draws attention to the finger and is used by some to highlight other things, such as the ring on the finger with the accent nail.

An accent nail looks as follows:

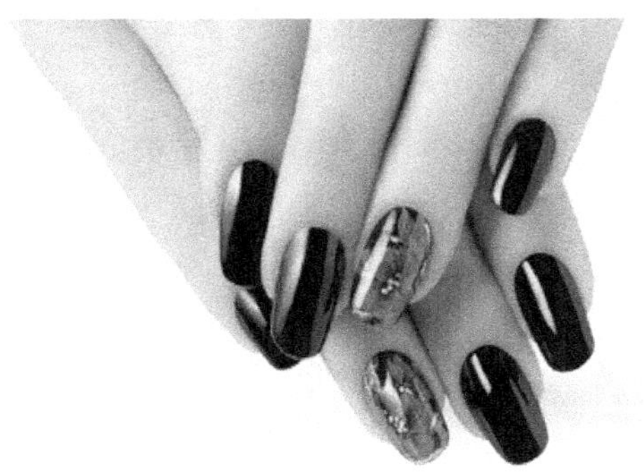

A beginner can always experiment on an accent nail and the rest of the nails can be designed as follows from simplest to the most complicated (still for beginners):

• Applied with base coat only for a shiny, natural look;

• Colored using nail polish (including the glittery kind) without any other designs;

● Designed using nail polish and nail art stickers by doing the following:

1. After applying the base coat and letting it dry, apply polish on the nail.
2. Let the polish dry before applying the nail art stickers.
3. Apply top coat.

● Designed using improvised nail art designs on a plastic sandwich bag instead of acrylic nails. As mentioned in *Chapter 4 What's Involved? Materials and Methods*, the use of acrylic nails may result to fungus infection, hence it is recommended that in case acrylic nails are really preferred by the wearer, then at least let the application be performed by a professional. Consider that any infection underneath the acrylic nails will most likely not be detected early unless the acrylic paint is used temporarily only.

To avoid the risk of infection entirely though, simply improvise using a plastic sandwich bag by doing the following:

1.   Apply base coat on nail and let it dry.

2. Apply nail polish on a plastic sandwich bag. Design nail polish as desired.

3. Peel the nail polish from the plastic. Apply nail glue on nail plate and press the designed polish on nail.

4.   Cut extra nail polish, if any

5. Apply top coat on the polish and ensure that the whole finger is covered including the edges.

6. This method would not provide the convenience of a ready-made acrylic nail, but it would at least be a very convenient venue for practicing nail accents, especially since it would be difficult to design nail art on one's own hands.

- Designed as glitter gradients using glitter nail polish and striping tape by doing the following:

1. After applying the base coat and letting it dry, apply polish on the nail.
2. Apply glitter nail polish on upper portion of the nail. Apply until the desired effect is achieved. Another glitter nail polish may also be applied.
3. Let the polish dry before applying the top coat.

- Designed as newspaper nails using polish, rubbing alcohol and newspaper clippings by doing the following:
1. After applying the base coat and letting it dry, apply light or nude polish on the nail.
2. Pour rubbing alcohol or water in a container. Note that the design may not be as clear if water was used.

3. Dip the nail in the rubbing alcohol or water for 5 seconds.

4. Press the newspaper clipping on your nail. Do this firmly and carefully peel the newspaper.

5. Apply top coat.

Letters may also be used as simple nail art designs with probable meaning.

• Designed as half-moon manicure using nail stickers and polish. Nail polish remover and brush may also be necessary to clean-up the manicure.

Do the following to create this effect:

1. After applying the base coat and letting it dry, place a French manicure sticker across the nail and leave the tip exposed. Ensure that the sticker is pressed down on the nail to avoid polish, as much as possible, from staining this part. Other stickers may also be used for this.
   Apply polish on the exposed part.

2. Remove the sticker before the nail polish has dried to avoid pulling off the paint along with the sticker.

3. Use nail polish remover and brush to clean up whatever polish had gone over the half-moon that the sticker should have prevented. This is one of those cases wherein the nail polish correction pen would be very handy. To avoid messing up the good part, let the polish dry a bit (but not completely) before removing the excess

4. Let the nail polish dry before applying the top coat.

5. Do the same to the rest of the nails

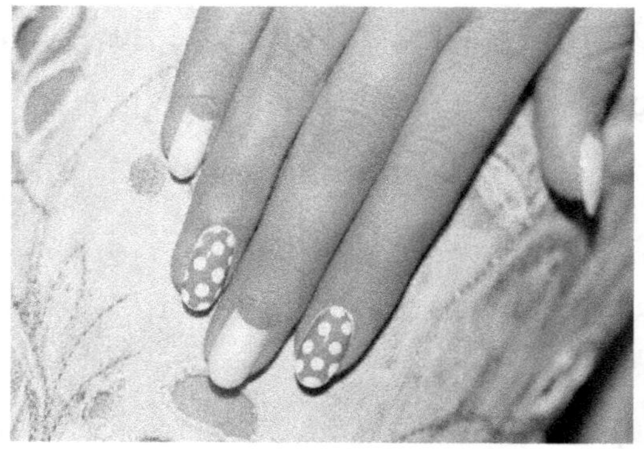

- Designed using stamping kits by doing the following:

1. After applying the base coat and letting it dry, apply the polish on the nail.

2. Apply a different polish on the desired design on the stamping template. It is recommended that the polish is thick and highly pigmented.

3. Use the scraper to remove the excess polish. Hold the scraper so that its angle would be at 45 degrees.

4. Use the stamper to collect the design from the template. Press firmly.

5. Stamp the design over the nail. Be careful in this step since it is necessary to be firm but there is also the possibility that the polish would be destroyed in this step if too much pressure was exerted.

6. Add nail polish to the template and repeat the process to create a more vivid effect,

if deemed necessary. If the polish was destroyed in the previous step, though, then there will be a need to repeat the procedure from the top after applying nail polish remover.

7.   Let the nail polish dry before applying the top coat.

8.   Make sure to clean the stamping tools after use.

•   Designed using dotting tools, which can produce different designs such as flowers, simplified Mickey Mouse, etc.

1.   After applying the base coat and letting it dry, apply polish on the nail.

2.   Dip dotting tool on a different polish and apply to nail. Different dotting tools with different sizes may be used for this activity.

Dotting tool/s may also be dipped in different nail polishes. Also make use of glitters if desired.

- Let the polish dry before applying the top coat

- Designed as Ombre nails using polish and makeup sponge by doing the following:

1. Apply petroleum jelly on the surrounding skin of the nail. This will make it easier to remove the polish that will most likely stain the skin.
2. Apply a base coat on the nail and let it dry.

3. Dip a makeup sponge in water and wring out most but not all of the water. Retain enough water to ensure that the sponge will not absorb the nail polish that will be applied on it. This step will also prevent the nail polish to dry up before being applied on the nail.

4.   Apply nail polish on the makeup sponge. Once satisfied, apply a different nail polish on the makeup sponge and so on.

5.   Press the makeup sponge on the nail. Dab and roll the sponge from side to side, repeatedly, until you are satisfied with the shade and the concentration of the nail polish, as well as its Ombre effect.

6.   Reapply more polish to the sponge as necessary.

7.   Let the polish dry before applying the top coat. Consider applying more top coat than usual to smoothen out the surface as much as possible.

8.   Use a brush dipped in polish remover to clean the surrounding skin.

Chapter 8: Advanced Nail Art Designs

There are various ways to step nail art up a notch. Some of these ways are indicated below, including the step-by-step guide on how to achieve these looks.

- **Create water-marbled effect.**

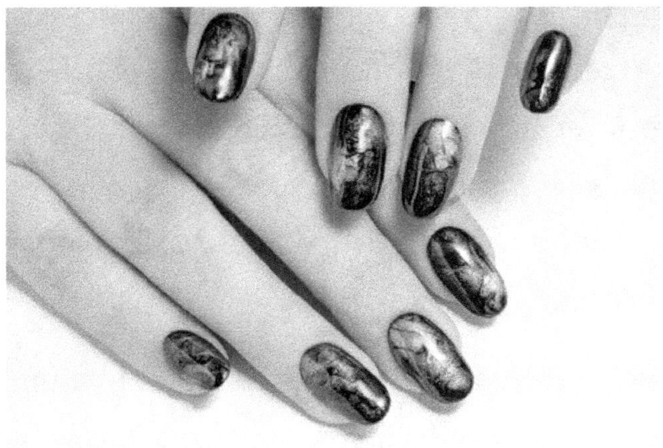

This could be created by doing the following:

1. After applying the base coat and letting it dry, pour water on a container.

2. Drop nail polish from a low height. The polish would create a circle on the water.

3.   Add another nail polish.
4. Use toothpick to create a design
5. Apply petroleum jelly on the nail/s and on the finger/s.
6. Slightly dip the nail/s on the solution
7. Clean up the manicure using nail polish remover. The nail correction pen would be very handy in this nail art method.
8. Allow the polish to dry before applying the top coat.

Design each nail differently, while maintaining a design for each nail that is harmonious with the rest. Think of the nails collectively instead of separately and create a design for each nail that should be related with the rest. It does not have to be that complicated. For example, nails may be colored brown.

For the two innermost nails, the eyes of a cat may be drawn whereas the ears may be drawn for the two next innermost nails. Nails may also be designed as per the pictures below.

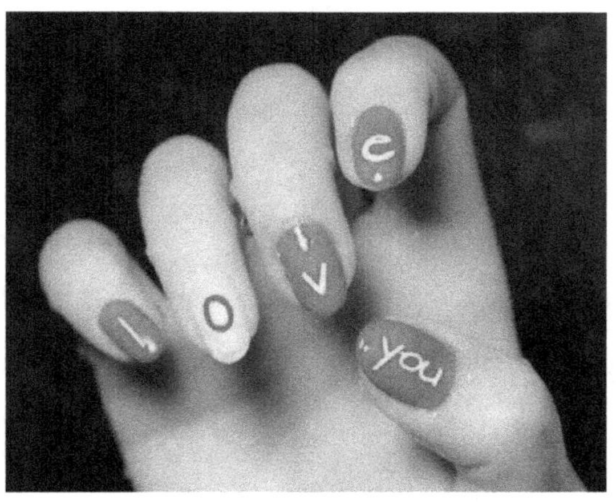

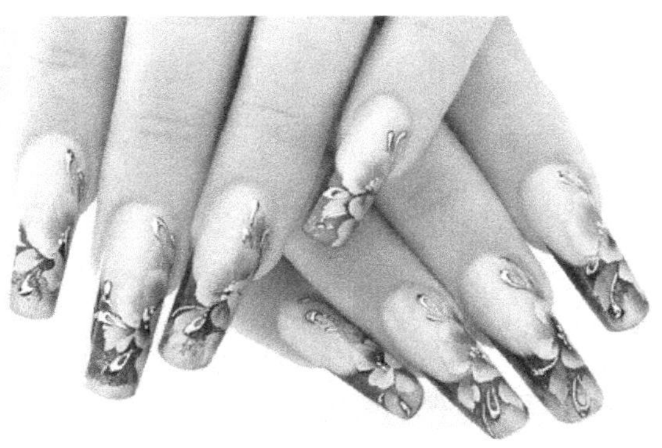

Chapter 9:   Additional Ideas & Designs

There are various ways to expand one's knowledge and skills on nail art. These are as follows:

•   Join an online community for nail art designs such as Nailpolis and Nail Nation. Be amazed at how artists could create different nail art designs. Be friendly with both newbies and experts. Learn from the mistakes and successes of others. Go beyond your comfort zone and never copy them but store knowledge of what could apply to you for later experimentations. Also take note of what you should avoid.

•   Famous nail art designs would also most likely be trending or shared on your social network, especially in Pinterest, so be on the look-out for these on your home page and even in your search bar, especially since even famous people are joining in on the fun.

Also consider looking for nail art designs that are seasonal, such as those that are Halloween or summer-themed for more unique ideas.

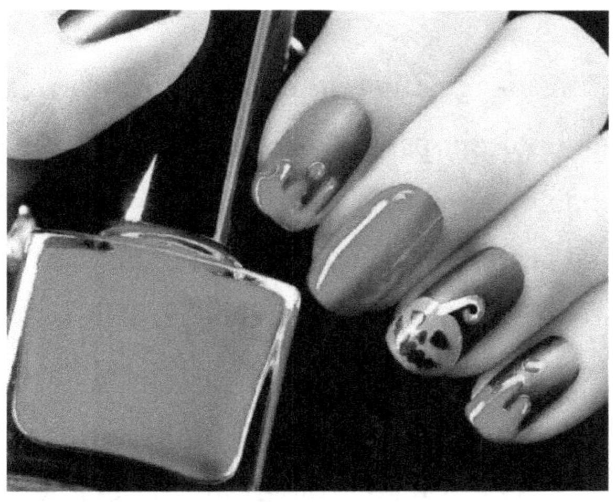

• Apart from these, nail art design can be researched in Google and other search engines. Different tips and methods are usually shared in personal blogs. Also check-out Style Caster for a list of the best blogs on nail art.

• It is also recommended to utilize the numerous online videos on nail art.

Videos are normally found in YouTube but so that your search will not be limited, use the Google search engine instead and videos from other websites would also appear.

• Consider reading other books by browsing online book shops. Read reviews before purchasing any book, the same way that reviews on nail art materials and tools should be read before the products are purchased. This is especially true if the products being sold are more expensive than the rest. Make sure that the products would be worth the price otherwise there are lots of others, including alternatives that may also provide the qualities needed.

If you feel more comfortable discussing ideas with someone face-to-face or to watch live instructions and performance instead of instructional videos, then you could also consider going to nail salons near you.

At salons, nail designers can advise what products work and what doesn't, as well as any other special tips that you might not otherwise get online. Formal lessons or classes can also be taken; albeit these may be expensive. You can always start getting the information online though. Search Google Maps for nail salons near you.

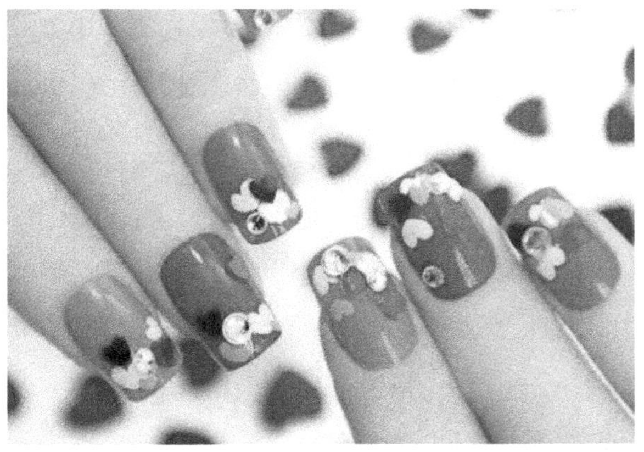

Chapter 10: Conclusion

With the amount of years spent by human civilization on developing nail art, it is no wonder that there are lots of things to explore. The potential for improvement is still there. What is important is to start small so as not to be overwhelmed. Try every variety of nail art materials and tools, while ensuring that your nails are not damaged. No product should be worth your nail.

There are various nail art designs online and tips from different people so do not settle for less in terms of quality. Then never limit yourself with what is written on the pages and on the cyber space. Experiment with every materials and tools available to get what you want and always remember that materials and tools can be store-bought but they don't necessarily have to be premade.

Any item or tool can aid you in your design. Just look back at the improvised nail art materials and tools enumerated in *Chapter 6 How to do Nail Art at Home – Step by Step* which could result to beautiful nail arts if done correctly.

Practice and understand current trends but learn to challenge them. You will surely create a design that you would and you should be proud of.

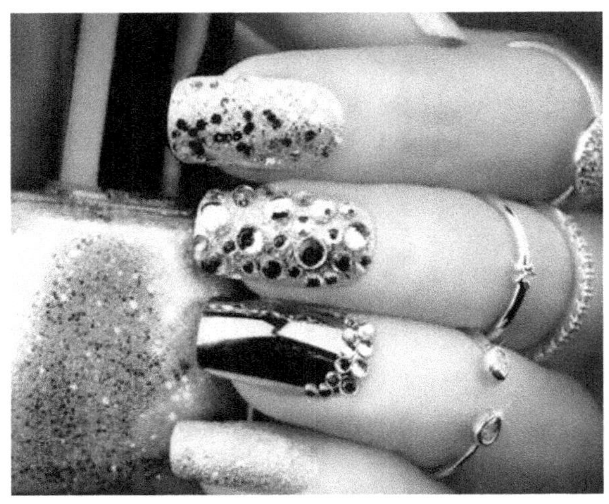

www.ingramcontent.com/pod-product-compliance
Lightning Source LLC
Chambersburg PA
CBHW060812260726
48660CB00002B/905